The New Equilibrium Diet

By Ike W. Sampson

Copyright © 2018 Ike W. Sampson

All Rights Reserved Worldwide

Contents

Introduction

Let's face it. You don't want to diet. You want to be at a new weight. It might be 10 pounds less. It might be 40. It doesn't matter. You just want it gone. Perhaps you've tried "The __________ Diet" or "The ___-_______ Diet". Or you've tried a "crash diet" – where you diet and then you crash. You pretty well know those don't work. Or you wouldn't be reading this book.

Equilibrium

What is "Equilibrium" anyway? Well, it is when everything is in balance. For example, when you ride in an airplane, the pilot climbs up to, say, 32,000 feet. The plane is cruising at 550 miles per hour. It stays there. Everything is smooth. The thrust of the jet engines is balanced against the drag caused by pushing it through the air. The lift of the wings is in balance with the weight of the plane. It is in equilibrium. So, how does this apply to you? Simple, if you have been 20 pounds overweight for the last 10 years, or even for the last 1 year, you are pretty much in equilibrium. That's good news. You are most of the way there! You are not gaining weight. Your eating and your activity are in balance. (Now, if you ARE gaining weight, then that is a different story. You should turn to

Chapter 5). Your caloric intake matches your body's need for energy. Your daily activities, plus the normal "operating needs" of your body are consuming the calories, or energy, you are putting into it on a daily basis. You are in equilibrium.

If you change the amount of food you consume, or if you change the metabolism of your body (like some diet pills do, by adding a stimulant into your system) or change the activities you do, you tip the balance out of equilibrium. You will gain weight. Or you will lose weight. It's not rocket science, as they say. (Ok, I'm not really sure who "they" are. But I am a rocket scientist.)

Now, if you are like most people, you gain weight as you get older. Why? Well a big reason is that your body slows down. What do I mean by that? I mean to say that your body's basic metabolism gets slower. I've seen it many times. I have worked with guys twenty to thirty years younger than I am. Often we have to share some particular computer, or if I'm out of my office, someone will sit in my chair to talk to my office mate. (Ok, it is only a cube, but office sounds more important.) And when I sit in a chair that was previously occupied by one of these guys, the chair is warm to me. They are burning more energy than I am. Just by sitting. Consequently, if you are eating the same amount of food over the years, unless you increase the activities you do, you will gain weight. Your body at idle burns less. In one way, that's good. You don't need as much food. But, that's not the way any of us think. I liked being able to eat as much pizza as I wanted, and not gain weight. Or get that double cheeseburger, large fries and a shake. I still want to do that. I can't, at least not very often.

In fact, it doesn't really take that much of a change over the years to put us on a long term weight gain. Think about this, if you consume an extra 10 calories a day (I think that is about 1 LifeSaver), over the course of a year, you will gain about a pound. (Using the formula 1 pound of fat = 4000 calories) 10 calories X 365 days in a year = 3650 calories. NOW (and this is the scary part), multiply this by 30 years, and voila, you are 30 pounds overweight. And you really haven't done anything. It was very gradual, very subtle. Maybe you are not eating much of anything more. Maybe your body is just slowing down by 10 calories a day. I think you typically burn around 2000 calories a day. All that has to happen is for your body to slow down to 1990 calories a day. A change of zero point five percent. This is so slight in comparison, it would hardly be noticeable. And it's not. Until 25 or 30 years later, you realize you aren't that trim 22 year old anymore that you remember.

Disclaimers

What?! A disclaimer? Yes, I really should say something terrific, and then put a tiny asterisk next to it (*), and then way at the back of the book, add in all the disclaimers, in very tiny print. But I'm not made that way. Let some other book do that. My healthcare provider sent out a healthy living and dieting guideline. The headline letters were 12 mm tall, and tucked away at the bottom, in tiny print (a little over 1 mm) was this disclaimer: "*The … program is … a voluntary weight loss program that is offered to eligible participants as part of their benefit plan. The information provided under this program is for general informational purposes only and is not intended to be nor should be construed as medical and/or nutritional advice. Participants should consult an appropriate health care professional to determine what may be right for them. …". Did you see that? *"not intended to be nor should be construed as medical and/or nutritional advice"*. That from a healthcare company, you know, one with doctors and hospitals. Hmmm.

The jump rope I purchased has this disclaimer on the box: "Note: As with any exercise product or program, use with caution and consult your physician prior to use."

SO, if these groups are disclaiming any responsibility for what they provide, who am I to do anything less? Here's my disclaimer: I invoke all the above disclaimers. Plus, use this program at your own risk. Consult your physician before using any of the guidelines stated in this book. I will not be responsible for any adverse effects from following this program. Exercise due caution in performing any of the activities mentioned in this book.

And a few more: If you or any of your IM forces are caught or killed, the secretary will disavow any knowledge of your actions. (from the original "Mission Impossible" television series). Your mileage may vary. It will probably be less. (from EPA car mileage ratings) Results not typical. (from the small print in a lot of television ads, especially late night TV)

With all that said, you may now proceed to continue with this book.

Scales and scales

GET a scale. Spend $20 and get a digital scale. Not an analog one. You might ask why. Then again, you might not. I'm going to tell you anyway. Here's why: an analog scale, unless it is one of those double beam ones with the sliding weights, is not going to give you the precision needed to tell you if anything is happening. A digital scale will usually give a readout to the two tenths of a pound. (the rest of the world uses kilograms) And it will read out to a tenth of a kilogram. And since a kilogram is about 2 pounds, ok 2.2, then a tenth of 2.2 rounds down to .2 pounds. That's how it is. It might not be accurate, but it is precise. If you weigh yourself at the same physiological time each day, then you will get a better idea of your progress. You will get more instantaneous feedback about the steps you take each day and how they affect your weight. Don't get carried away, however. An eight ounce cup of coffee, once you drink it, will cause you to weigh half a pound more. So depending on time of day, meal size, when you expel liquids and solids, your weight might vary by three pounds in a given day. It is important, then to choose a time of day that will consistently represent you. The morning, after a visit to the bathroom is usually a good time. Some things to remember, or at least keep in mind. If you're like me, one day to the next is not without some randomness. My solid waste disposal cycle is not daily. It varies from two to three day intervals. Liquid is pretty consistent. I can outlast most of my peers, when it comes to long and boring meetings….even when I'm drinking coffee. (There's a Dilbert cartoon relating to this.)

Eating Less

I know this may come as a shock, but part of the equation is what you eat. Or more correctly, how much you eat, and how many calories the food has. What is a calorie, anyway? It is a unit of energy. Your body needs energy. And if your body finds it has more energy available than it needs, it stores the energy, as fat. It's not rocket science. And if it gets less energy than it needs, it takes that fat and "burns" it to get the energy it needs. Yes, a dietitian will give you a better, and more detailed analysis. If you have fat, then you want to eat a little less than you have been eating, or more to the point, you want less calories. There are lots of simple ways to do this, without "going on a diet". Let's look at some:

You are part of a Friday donut club. You've been doing this for years. No, I'm not even going to suggest that you stop. Here's what to do: When you get your donut, and after you take that first bite, break off a piece of it, AND THROW IT AWAY. And now, enjoy the rest of your donut. Trust me, you will never miss the part you threw away. But you just knocked off a hundred calories, more or less, from your daily intake. 100 x 52 weeks is almost a pound and a half over the course of a year. (4000 calories = 1 pound of fat). Remember, you got to your heavyweight condition over the course of a number of years, with the addition of little things like this, so you can just as easily send the scale in the other direction.

You like your Snickers ™ bar every afternoon with your coffee. (I think you already know what I am about to tell you...) Unwrap it, break off a small piece of it, AND THROW IT AWAY. Then, enjoy your Snickers ™. Last I checked, Snickers ™ is about 300 calories. You just threw away 50 of them. 50 calories x 52 weeks x 5 days a week = 13,000 calories. Or just over 3 pounds of fat.

In the morning, you enjoy a glass of good old Florida fresh (not from concentrate) orange juice. It's great! No, I'm not going to ask you to spit out your first gulp of it. How about on Tuesdays and Thursdays, have a glass of V-8 ™ instead? Or pure tomato juice? Or your store's generic version. Orange juice: 110 calories. V-8 ™: 40 calories. A savings of 70 calories a serving x 2 days a week x 52 weeks = 7280 calories, or just under 2 pounds of stored energy. (You thought I would say "fat", didn't you?)

Or, if you really don't like V-8 ™, or even V-9, then try this on for size: First pour a half glass of good old fashioned WATER. Once you have finished that, then pour yourself a half glass of orange juice and finish out your breakfast with that. 55 calories saved. And you get the great taste of orange juice lingering in your mouth.

Do you like peanuts? I know I do. I can't really tell you how much a handful of peanuts is, but I know that I get just as much enjoyment out of a half handful of peanuts as I do a full handful. It takes some effort to pour a little less into my hand, but I think it cuts about 50 or so calories, maybe more. And I probably have some peanuts twice a day. So, you know the drill: 50 calories x 2 times a day x 5 days a week x 52 weeks = YIKES, 26,000 calories, or 6 ½ pounds of stored energy. Wow, until just now, I didn't realize just how a little thing like peanuts can add up.

Another thing you can do is put a bag of baby carrots in the door of the refrigerator. Or baby celery. Good munching material. Especially if you have some hummus around. Hummus is one of those touted superfoods. And it comes in many very tasty varieties. Carrots and celery are just about calorie-less. Hummus is a lot lower in calories than any chip dip, unless you dip your chips in hummus. Anyway, chips are not a good thing (and donuts are?), and if you can break yourself from chips and dip while watching soap operas, then you are a leg up. I understand that snacking on celery is a zero cost option: the stick of celery has about one calorie, and it takes one calorie of energy to eat it. Now, here's where it gets dangerous. Dip that celery in peanut butter, and suddenly you have a

hundred calories on that celery: Peanut Butter is 100 calories per

tablespoon. Or dip that celery in Ranch Dressing, and you have 130

calories per tablespoon. But dip it in some mustard, and you have a

winner. There are two mustard containers in my fridge: Heinz Organic

Yellow Mustard, and Boar's Head Delicatessen Style Mustard. Each is

ZERO calories per tablespoon. (Others are about 5. Some can be up to

80....your mustard may vary.)

Again, carrots are about 175 calories per pound. Get a pound of

baby carrots, put the bag in the door of the fridge. OPEN THE BAG. That is

the only way you will opt for them as a snack over something more

calorie loaded. You will be 2.7 times more like to grab a couple of carrots

if the bag is open and at eye level. They make a quick snack, and satisfy

your urge to chew on something. If you don't like mustard, hummus

makes a VERY tasty dip, and is 50 calories for two tablespoons. That's ¼

the calories of peanut butter. It comes in many flavors, too.

Do you pack a lunch? One sandwich or two? Here's what to do.

On one sandwich, use only one slice of bread. Yes, put the whole

sandwich worth of fixings into a half slice of bread, and cap it off with the

other half slice. You just saved 100 calories. Times 5 days a week. Times

50 weeks a year. (I'm giving you two weeks of vacation.) That equals

25,000 calories, or 6 and a quarter pounds.

How about breakfast? Do you have two biscuits of shredded

wheat? A few times a week, break one biscuit in two, and have one and a

half biscuits for breakfast. It is a savings of 40 calories and you'll probably

never notice. Change that milk to almond milk, and you go from 110

calories to 40, per whatever they call a "serving".

While I am not a fan of soft drinks, you might be. Unless you are

one of those people they put on the commercials who can taste the

difference between Coke ® and Pepsi ®, then you could easily switch to

the diet version of whatever sugar-laden soft drink you now consume,

and knock off about 110 calories a serving. Let's assume you have one

soft drink a day at work. 110 calories x 5 days x 52 weeks = 28,600

calories, or just over 7 pounds of stored energy.

I haven't totaled the annual savings of the above minor changes,

but I'm guessing it adds up (or subtracts down) to around 30 pounds. IN

ONE YEAR. WITHOUT DIETING. Your mileage may vary. You can certainly

think of many more just as clever little changes that you could do. So do them. Just "Nudge" them into your routine, and you will be on your way,

gently, to that lower weight that you have in mind.

Exercising More

There are a lot of little things you can do in your day to burn just a few more calories…it doesn't take any more time. You don't have to join a "gym" or fitness center. Here are just a few of the many things you can do:

- Run in place while your coffee is brewing in the morning. Yes, it is that simple. I turn on the espresso machine and make some café Americano to go, every morning. The whole process is about 90 seconds. While the machine is running, I can easily run in place about 150 steps. It boosts my heart rate moderately. I do something besides stand there watching the cup fill. It doesn't take me any longer to get out the door.

- Do some sit-ups. If you have a bed with a footboard, you can probably do 20 sit-ups before you even get out of bed. I do. I just hook my feet under a part of the footboard, and the mattress is a great cushion. It beats doing sit-ups on the floor. It takes about 30 or 40 seconds. Unless you slam your body back into the mattress after each sit-up, you probably won't even awaken your spouse.

- Jumping jacks. Yes, those things. You remember them, right? Gym class, from 1st grade on. 100 jumping jacks don't take more than 2 minutes. Do them anywhere. No tools required.

- If you are really gutsy, buy a $6 jump rope. Do this in the garage. TRY to jump 100 times. I know, the kids in high school can jump 100 times in about 10 seconds. In fact, I think somebody at my kids' high school recorded 136 jumps in 10 seconds. It looked like he was standing inside a running jet engine. You and I aren't usually so nimble. Plus, if you miss…well that puts a real slowdown on things. Three minutes of jump roping is more than I can take. Really! I'll be dripping with sweat and exhausted. So, set a goal for a measly 3 minutes every day. If you can do that, then WOW! If not, well neither can I. But give it a try. Boxers do it. They can't be wrong, can they?

- Toe lifts. Ok, you are not lifting your toes. You are lifting with your toes. In other words, lift your heels off the ground, as high as you can, while you are standing. So you will be standing on tip-toes. You can do this anywhere. (Ok, you probably don't want to do this in a crowd of people. They will start to look at you funny.) Go up and down. 60 times in less than a minute is a pretty good pace. This does more than you think. The muscles you use are very strong ones. They are used to lifting you all day long. More than likely, this will be easy. You won't even get tired. But think about it – a lot of work is being done. If you weigh 200 pounds, you are lifting 200 pounds about 3 inches off the ground. Times 60. That comes out to 3,000 foot-pounds of work. That is the equivalent of lifting your car a foot off the ground.

-   "Almost" push-ups. I call them push-outs. Ok, if you want to, drop to the floor and do 20 push-ups. But if that doesn't appeal to you, do some almost push-ups. Find a wide hall-way, or maybe the space between your bed and your dresser. About 4 or 4 ½ feet will do nicely. Now lean into the dresser, or wall or bathroom vanity, and hold yourself by your outstretched arms. Scoot or place your feet against the bed, or wall or the bathtub, or, or, or. You are probably at a 45 degree angle. Now, do the push-ups. Start with 10 if you have to. 20 shouldn't be hard. Keep your body straight. It doesn't help to bow your body in. That's cheating. There's no point to cheating – you just cheat yourself. The advantage is that this is less weight to lift, and you don't have to get down on the floor. And again, it doesn't take that much time. You can do it in passing, perhaps even a few times a day, if you have it in you to do so.

- Trunk twists. Again, like the toe-lifts, you will probably get funny looks if you do this in a crowd. Stand straight. Hold your arms straight out, to the side. Then, using an eight count. Twist 45 degrees to the right. Then another 45. (That's about as far as most of us can go. If you can go a third 45, my hat's off to you. If you are one of those Romanian gymnasts, you can probably twist a full circle without any problems at all. But then again, if you are one of those Romanian gymnasts, you probably aren't reading this book.) Where was I? Oh. Now on the third count, twist to the left 45 degrees, then back straight. Then 45 degrees to the left, then another 45. Then to the right 45. Then back to straight. If you did all this correctly, it will be 8 counts, and you are back to center. All the time, keep your arms straight out, to the side. Don't beat yourself up with this. 10 reps is a good number.

- Squats. You remember these from gym class as well. Hold your arms straight in front of you, at shoulder level. Then just lower your body by bending your knees. If you are a dancer type, you will know that you need to keep your back straight. And THAT, is hard. If you are not a dancer, you will just do this in any old fashion, and for the purpose of getting your body to do some work, that will be just fine. 10 squats is a good number.

- Lastly, (well maybe not), toe touching. Can you even do that? It was easy as a kid. I could put my whole palm flat on the ground. Now, I lucky to barely touch my toes with the tips of my fingers. Try for 10 of these. Good stretching, even you can only come close to your toes. Hey, if in the NFL, you can just wave a part of your body, or the football, over the plane of the goal and it's a touchdown, then I think that if you just get close to your toes it still counts.

- When you go to a store, park in the farthest parking space. And WALK. Walking is a good thing. Caveat this: if it's snowing or raining, maybe you should use your own discretion. Also, if you have little ones, then never mind. Find the closest space.

You don't need the aggravation of trying to navigate any farther than you have to with little ones. Plus, it is a safety issue, with little ones and parking lots. (That's partly because parking lots are designed ALL WRONG, but don't get me started on that. I'll save it for a different book.)

- While you are at the store, start by going to the farthest corner of the store, before you even start to look for the things you need. And then, especially in a grocery store, walk up and down every aisle, even if you came for just a couple of things. You will have burned just that many more calories. One, you might see things you need. Two, you will get a pretty good walk. It doesn't take that long. Unless you go to one of those COSTCO super stores, or the other guy super stores. (I don't like the other guy, so I won't mention its name.)

- What can you do at your desk? Push down on the desktop. Lift your legs out straight. Lift up from under your desktop (as long as nobody stuck bubble gum there…). Put your hands on the arms of the chair and press in. Do the same with your elbows. Then pull out with your hands. Push out with your elbows. Try to lift yourself off the chair, pushing upwards on the seat with your hands. Now do it using the armrests. ONE BIG CAVEAT: make sure the chair is sturdy enough to do this.

- What can you do while you are driving? Pull the steering wheel towards you. Push it away from you. Pull left with your left hand, while pulling right with your right hand. Then push the sides of the steering wheel towards the center. ONE BIG CAVEAT: make sure you can do this safely while you are driving.

- Get your 10 cents worth. Another place you should walk is around your house. Devise a route that takes you into and out of every room in the house. Put 10 pennies at one end of the route. Your goal is to move those pennies from one end of your route to the other, every day. NO, you can't pick up ALL the pennies at once. Only one at a time, please. Make sure you touch (or come close to) every window and door in the house. That adds to your walk. This way you get a good walk in without having to brave any bad weather. If there are stairs, so much the better. If you have an elevator, try not to use it unless you have to.

- If you can, work in walking a mile every day. Twenty minutes is about right if you walk briskly. (You might have gotten in a mile going to Costco ™...) Here's the deal: I'm told that walking or running a mile burns about 100 calories. And some residual, as it boosts your metabolism for an hour or two. PRINT THIS INDELIBLY INTO YOUR HEAD. Because, when you pick up that cheeseburger, or milk shake, or whatever your most tempting snack is, figure out how many calories it is, then think about how many miles of walking that you will have to do to counter-balance those calories. If you are a normal person, you will start gauging the enjoyment of the food vs the number of miles of walking it represents.

- But while I'm on this subject, wrap your brain around this: if you do nothing else but add walking a mile a day to your routine (about 20 minutes), you will burn 36,500 extra calories every year, which is about 9 pounds of stored energy. So, in a little over 4 years (about 4 ½) , you could take off all those 40 pounds you have put on in the last 25 or 30 years. That's how easy this is.

- Now, if you want to lose 60 pounds in a year, go read somebody else's book. There are plenty of them out there. However comma the point here is to make a gentle nudge in how you do things so that you don't feel deprived, and so you don't "backslide". Remember this is not about the act of losing weight, but it is about gradually becoming you with 40 pounds less and doing it so that you establish that as a new equilibrium at that lower weight.

Building Muscle (Boosting your metabolic rate)

I've read that your body consumes more calories, even at rest, if you have more muscle. So, if over the course of a day, your resting body burns 30 or 40 more calories, then that's a good thing. Because it's work you don't have to do. Let's face it. Over the years, many of us (ok, ME) have gotten less muscular, less active. If you see a set of barbells, dumbbells, or cowbells for that matter, buy a set. Do some curls, squats, lifts, or even hold these things out to the side at shoulder level. Read up on what protein helps you build muscle. My favorite is prime rib.

But, I'm not putting a lot of emphasis on this particular aspect of nudging. You may not like to go to a gym. Or run marathons, or be able to press 350 pounds. It is just one more tool to consider. There are numerous books and fitness centers around that are more versed in muscle-building than I am.

Lead us Not into Temptation

Suddenly, you are not going to snack – Sure! Most of us tend to snack. It's ok. You have maintained your weight (sort of), and snacked. Still, here's another place that you can exercise some good judgment, before you are ready for a snack, and shave off another little bit. It works like this: you will snack on whatever you have. If you have chips and dip in the house, you will eat it. If you have crackers and brie cheese (a favorite of mine), you will eat that. There is no debate. There is no soul searching. You are hungry! You are NOT going to look in the cupboard, past the microwave packet of buttered popcorn, and say to yourself, "I guess I'll have to go to the store. I need to chew on some celery." I don't blame you. It's not "You are what you eat." It's "You eat what you have."

To make sure you have what you won't feel badly about later, make the choice when you write out your shopping list, or at least when you are in the store. If you bring home baby carrots and hummus, then when you get the snack urge, you will eat baby carrots and hummus. Decide for yourself what you want to have on hand for a reasonably healthy, tasty, and non-high caloric snack. Pick up boxes at the store and read the labels. Carefully. Some snacks quote a calorie count, per serving, that sounds pretty good, until you look at the clever sleight of hand:

serving size. Some candy bars have a serving size of ½ the candy bar. Get real! If I get a Snickers from a vending machine at work, I am not going to eat just half, and put the other half away for tomorrow.

Seasonal Gravity Anomaly

You've never heard of it, right? Well, have you heard of the South Atlantic Anomaly? No, huh?

Ok, if you are a rocket scientist type, you would have. But, for the rest of you, The South Atlantic Anomaly is an area, in ….. the South Atlantic, where the Van Allen radiation belts dip closer to the earth. Why is this important? It's important because some satellites, depending on their inclination, perigee, right ascension, etc, could pass through this regularly, and it can affect the electronics of the satellite. Almost always in a bad way.

The Seasonal Gravity Anomaly is like that, too. If you are in North America, specifically the U. S., you pass through the Seasonal Gravity Anomaly yearly. It starts about November 1st, has high points on the 4th Thursday of November, the 25th of December, 31st of December, the day of the Super Bowl, February 14th, and MardiGras. Yes, all that celebrating, along with extra eats, causes gravity to increase in humans, as indicated by stepping on the scale and discovering that gravity has increased by 5, 10, or even 20 pounds. If you work in an office, it starts when leftover Halloween candy is brought in. And then the whole month of December is a mine field. Happy co-workers bring in cookies, fudge, cake, and candy canes. And you have to be polite and have some. It would be rude to always say "No thanks." Oh, and did I mention the company "Winter Holiday" Party? Yeah, nobody is allowed to say "Christmas" anymore. But just what Winter Holiday is being celebrated, if not Christmas? I'll leave that as an exercise to the reader. Your friends will also have Christmas parties and dinners and such. (They can at least say "Christmas".)

But back to the main point: it is easy to undo a lot of your efforts during the Seasonal Gravity Anomaly. I realize that you've been through it before, and will continue to do so year after year. Satellites that go through the South Atlantic Anomaly are built with extra shielding, now that they know that it exists. (I suspect that a lot of the earlier satellites weren't so fortunate.) And now that you know, build in some extra shielding into your routine as you go through the Seasonal Gravity Anomaly. Because you will go through the Seasonal Gravity Anomaly EVERY year for the rest of your life.

How to do build that extra shielding? Plan ahead. Work out some phrases, such as "Oh, I just had my lunch." "I still haven't finished the fudge that Debbie gave me yesterday." "Thanks, but I have to go to a big dinner tonight." Do you have to turn down EVERYTHING? Of course, not.

You didn't last year, and you did ok. Or, has the Seasonal Gravity

Anomaly, year after year, been the cause of the 30 or 40 extra pounds

you now carry around. Think a little. Gain two or three pounds each year.

Times how many years? It really doesn't take that much to get you where

you are today.

What about parties? They are great. Drinking at parties – not so

great. Two reasons: 1) if you are driving. 2) the alcohol is probably free. I

don't know about you, but if something is free, I tend to take advantage

of that. A good tack is to get some soda water with a lime in it. It looks

fancy, like a drink, and it is pretty tasty. Or, well I don't know what the

"Or" is. You will have to think of something.

Are you Comfortable in Your Skin?

Are you comfortable in your skin? Probably. Don't get too comfortable. Yes, you feel pretty ok in your current "skin". However, it's not the skin you want, is it? Otherwise, why are you reading this book? Consequently, be aware of this hindrance. As you begin to move towards your desired weight, you may feel a little uncomfortable. Clothes start to feel a little loose.

Do you weigh a pound more than last time? Live with it. "A pint's a pound, the world around." So goes the time-worn phrase. So when you weigh yourself, consider that fact. If you just drank a 12 oz. soft drink, you will weigh ¾ of a pound more. You should know that your weight fluctuates. In a given day you could easily weigh a pound or two more or less. Don't over-react. Look at the long term direction that you are taking. Just keep nudging.

Clean Your Plate?

Were you raised by depression era parents? If so, (or even if not) you may have been told, "You may not be excused until you finish all the food on your plate." That was the rule in my home. That plate had to be clean. It didn't matter what the meal was. It didn't matter if I liked it or not. Of course, it was worse if it was something I didn't like, like lima beans, or curried shrimp. Or peas, or asparagus. Or liver. And the tag line was "Think of the poor starving children in China." I succumbed. I tried several ways to hide peas under the plate, or in my napkin, but usually got caught. My brother, was a lot more clever (he told me later...) He'd fill his mouth with the offending food and get excused. Then he'd go up to the bathroom and spit it out. One day, after getting the tag line about the poor starving children in China, he pushed his plate away and said, "Ok, here. Give them this." I don't recall what happened next...

The point is, you don't have to clean your plate at every meal. In fact, in some cultures, the host is embarrassed if a guest cleans his plate. It implies that the host hasn't supplied enough food. Think of the cultural battle that would occur if the guest has been taught to clean his plate, and the host has been taught to keep refilling the food until the guest is full and leaves some food on the plate. It could really be funny if you have

the right sense of humor.

I Don't Have Time to Exercise

Really? Who told you to say that? If your day is really so busy...well let's see. Do you have time to make a cup of coffee? Yes? Then you have time to do 20 push-outs. Or 10 touch your toes. (Or "get close to" your toes.) Do you have time to wait for the water in your shower to warm up before you jump in? Yes? Then you have time to do 20 sit-ups. Or a hundred jumping jacks. Oh, I see. You have one of those new-fangled "instant" hot water heaters, so the moment you turn on the shower, it is hot. Ok, then you get a pass on that piece of time. BUT, Do you ever stop at a red light? Yes? Then you have time to do some steering wheel crunches. Or some leg-lifts (Put the car in PARK first. Or neutral with the parking brake on.) How about that? You really do have some time during the day. What a surprise...

However, that is not the way to look at it. This is an equation, after all. As you eat during the day, it is better to think of your "marginal" food in terms of their time cost to burn off those calories that you so casually consume. Remember the slice of bread I suggested you not eat? It is the equivalent to walking a mile. So, it is worth about 20 minutes. That one fifth of the candy bar came to about 50 calories, or about 10 minutes of walking. That handful of nuts: about 30 minutes of walking.

YES. I think you are starting to see this taking shape. What you don't have time for is that smidgeon of extra food that you really eat out of habit rather than need. Now, I am not suggesting that you take drastic measures to starve yourself. That will only backfire on you later. Remember, the title of this book is NUDGE. There are so many instances throughout the day, and you can take advantage of a few of them. The more you equate your intake with the equivalent work needed to burn off those calories, the better your mindset will become. Nobody will be keeping tabs on you. You will start making those decisions on your own. You will, won't you?! Yes, of course you will. You have a goal in mind. You have the means of reaching it. You are ok at arithmetic. This is not rocket science, as they say. Who are "they"? Nobody really knows. Well, at least, I don't.

A story relating to airplanes:

Years ago, when I was a young engineer, working for Boeing (don't get ahead of me – I worked on a rocket, not an airplane) I traveled regularly for monthly meetings. One day, I missed my 5 o'clock flight and had to catch a late evening one. The plane was barely half full. I had an aisle seat, the seat next to me was empty, and the window seat was occupied by a weary looking older gentleman, with a tattered brown valise at his feet. He was in a rumpled suit, and looked like the stereotypical traveling salesman. (I'm thinking "Willy Lowman" in Death of a Salesman). The plane took off, and headed over the Sierra Nevada mountain range. The seat belt sign was on. Only the stewardesses were moving around. (Yes, it was awhile ago. They were called stewardesses then. They were always female, young, slender, and attractive. Their hair was done up nicely, and they wore snug, but not tight, skirts, reaching just below the knees) As one of the stews was walking past me, towards the back of the plane, we suddenly hit a huge air pocket. She somehow bounced and landed in my lap, her arms around my neck. Apparently, I had instinctive wrapped my arms around her as well, to stop her fall. There we were, face to face, both completely stunned, looking at each other, for what seemed liked minutes, as the plane bounced around. Neither of us said a word. Then, as quickly as the whole thing started, the turbulence subsided. The young lady released her grip, (as did I. I think I helped her get upright, but I was still kind of in shock), got up, said a polite "Excuse me", straightened her skirt, and continued down the aisle. I just sat there, still bewildered at this chain of events, sort of cocooned by the noise of the jet. A minute or so later, I noticed out of the corner of my eye, the gentleman who was in the window seat, turning towards me.

With what seemed to be a mixture or lament and envy, he spoke, "I've been traveling for 35 years and nothing like that has ever happened to me."

What does that have to do with you getting down to your weight goal? Not a thing. Just thought it might amuse you. I remember that event fondly, and take great delight in retelling it.

Seven and a half cents

There is an old movie called "The Pajama Game", starring Doris Day and John Raitt. Alongside the obvious romantic tone of the movie, union garment workers are pushing for a 7 ½ cent per hour raise. At a rally for their cause, they sing (it's a musical) a song reflecting on how this meager increase in wages will affect their future. In one year …, in FIVE years…, in TEN years…, well you get the picture. If you get the chance, watch the movie and listen to the song. (ok, the song is near the end of the movie, so if you don't like musicals, you can fast forward). It has significant relevance here. Seven and a half cents is pretty insignificant. But, a year's worth (about 2088 hours) starts to mean something (approximately $156). And five years of increased wages really adds up: $783.

EVERY NUDGE you do works the same way. Each little nudge doesn't mean much, standing alone. But, if you gently keep it up, over the course of a year, it actually does stuff. And in a couple of years, should you need to take that long, Voila! You are there. You didn't diet. There's no diet to ruin. You didn't torture yourself with terrible foods. You arrive and you have an arsenal of methods to stay at your desired weight – at the new equilibrium. You did it gently and mostly unnoticed, by you or by anybody else.

Ok, this is another diversion, and it involves airplanes (again). The most enjoyable flight I've ever experienced was a 1 am "positioning" flight, from NYC's JFK airport to Atlanta. It was on a Lockheed L-1011, which is a huge airplane. It competed with the DC-10 and Boeing 747. This was back before deregulation, and all the price juggling that goes on today. Anyway, there were about 12 of us passengers. The "stewardesses" said to pick anywhere to sit. (There were about 300 seats in this cavernous airplane.) After take-off, they brought pillows and blankets, and we each took a row of seats and bedded down. There was nobody within 5 rows of my spot. I slept great! And about 30 minutes before landing, a stewardess awakened me with coffee, orange juice, and a hot breakfast. Yes, really! I think it was pancakes, sausage, scrambled eggs. And I'm pretty sure there was a hot towel somewhere in the mix as well. Those were the days...

Living Backwards Like Merlin

Do you remember the Disney movie "The Sword in the Stone"? One of the characters was the wizard "Merlin". According to the story, he lived backwards. The reason he knew the future was that he lived backwards through time. His past was (or is, or will be… it can be quite confusing) our future. At any rate, he got younger instead of getting older.

With that in mind, you should start living backwards, too. As you progress DOWN the weight scale, think of how old you were when you last were at that weight. (I'm assuming you were the lightest when you were born, and got heavier as time went forward. I hope that is a true statement.) You could hit ZZZ pounds and think, "WOW! I was at this weight when I lived in Sioux Falls, working as the area manager, 10 years ago." Or maybe you hit the weight you last had in your 20's. And then what you weighed when you got married. (Yes, I'm making a generalization here. Or maybe it was when you got divorced…) And then, you reach the weight you had when you graduated from college or high school. Actually, I wouldn't want to weigh what I weighed in high school and college. I was pretty skinny. I had a lot of "bread and air" sandwiches in college. That was all I could afford. (I actually managed to pay for college by working summers and on Saturdays during the school year. It would be very hard to do that today, with the price of college being what it is now.)

Celebrate these road signs! You've heard it said, "You're not getting any younger." Well, that is simply not true. You will be getting younger. Where you want your destination to be is entirely up to you. It is a pretty nice adventure.

Are You What You Eat?

Yes, I briefly addressed this before. It's worth going over again.
You have probably heard the phrase, "You are what you eat." I don't
know if that is true – probably is. But, I have a different phrase for you to
think about: "You eat what you have." AND, if you have it in bulk, you will
probably eat it in bulk. Let me give you an example. If you grocery shop
weekly, and buy a six-pack of beer, then you will probably have ONE beer
each evening with dinner. But if you buy a 12 pack or an 18 pack, or a
case of 24, then you will easily slide into having two beers each evening,
and maybe three on Saturday. (After all, that yard work made you pretty
thirsty. And nothing works to quench your thirst like a nice cold beer.) Ok,
you're more sophisticated than that. You drink wine. Instead of a 750ml
bottle of wine, you buy a 1.5 liter bottle of wine. So, at dinner, you say to
yourself, "there's a lot left. Look, it's not even a quarter empty.", and you
have a second glass. You wouldn't have done that if you had bought the
750ml bottle. And about that 2 pound jar of peanuts. It was a great deal
at Costco, wasn't it? Buying a 10 oz jar at the local grocery is more
expensive. However, You are going to take bigger and more handfuls
from that huge 2 pound jar. It isn't rocket science. This is just human
nature. It's my human nature, too. There aren't too many of us who are

immune. McDonald's wants us to "Super-Size" it. Burger King touts its

burger as a "Whopper". Carls Jr. advertises the "Six Dollar Burger" for just

$3.95.

Engineering 101

Another visit to the world of engineering: Trade Study or an Analysis of Alternatives. Or from the world of Economics, Net Present Value. This is a way to determine the most cost effective course of action. Perhaps you are building something, or designing a piece of equipment. There may be several ways of doing that. Each method is broken down into the parts and steps needed, and compared with the other ways of doing the job. Hopefully, the least costly way becomes clear. It is the same way with Nudge. You can cut a few things from your diet. Alternatively, you can add exercise to your day. Or you can do a little of both. Decide for yourself what method helps you achieve your goal the most efficient way. For example, you might skip that second slice of cheese on your lunch sandwich, saving 80 calories. How much effort does that take? Or, you could walk 8/10 of a mile, which would burn about 80 calories. It takes 15 to 20 minutes. Is it worth it to you to have the slice, or is it worth more to you to NOT have to walk for 15 to 20 minutes? That's really what it is, after the smoke clears.

Sprints

A sprint is a short duration run. In software development terms, it is a short period of time during which a particular objective is to be reached. Maybe there is a new feature to be added, or a screen interface to be changed, or who knows what. But the idea is to focus, for a short time (2-4 weeks, usually) on achieving that ONE thing.

How does this work in your world? It's like this. Perhaps at the beginning of the week you weigh 211.2 pounds. You set a goal of reaching 210.0 by the end of the week. So, for the next 4 days, you work on eating light, maybe even AVOIDING that tasty Friday doughnut. If you have wine with dinner, don't have any wine on Tuesday or Thursday. And you add a brisk 15 minute walk EVERY evening. Just for the week. To reach that ONE goal: 210.0 pounds. TaDa! I'll bet you dollars to doughnuts (bad example, I know) that you make it. Now, don't celebrate by ordering a large, stuffed crust, three-meat and three-cheese pizza. But make a mental note that you really did it. Mark it on the calendar.

Ok, sprint is over. Do this only once in a while. Not more than one time in a given month. And not for more than 3 or 4 days. It is a sprint, not a marathon. The result, however, is a good one. You've just crossed

off one of those pounds (or in this example, 1.2 pounds)

The Kid

What about the kid? There is a movie, starring Bruce Willis, called "The Kid". Through some mysterious happenings, he encounters his younger, child self, a pudgy, kid. He forgets to feed his younger self any breakfast, and so the kid is complaining. Bruce's assistant berates him for his negligence, at such time Bruce comments, "He could afford to skip a meal", in reference to the fact that the kid is pretty overweight.

Could you afford to skip a meal – just once in a while? Most of the world doesn't have the luxury of eating three meals a day, and snacks besides. A midnight snack is not even part of the vocabulary. We in America have huge refrigerators, stores that are open 24 hours a day, fast food and "fresh food fast" restaurants dotting the landscape, many of which are also open 24 hours a day. Is it possible that you could skip lunch tomorrow without withering away? Ok, maybe have a granola bar to tide you over. Go back to your regular lunches the following day. Or a dinner. You could have a big bowl of chunky soup instead. Some of them, even if you eat both servings (a can is usually two servings), it could be only 200 calories total.

Count Calories Because Calories Count

You've probably read lots of diet books that want you to ignore calories, and focus on carbohydrates, or fats, or what kinds of foods work well with other kinds of foods. Those are great ideas, sort of. The bottom line is not that complicated. Calories Count. Calories are the measure of the energy content of the food. And if you don't use the energy, your body stores it as ---- ok I'm going to say that word again --- FAT. In case you haven't noticed, a good number of people in the first world, particularly in the United States, and very particularly in some states, are FAT. They are not heavy with extra muscle, they are obese with FAT. I moved from one of the fittest states, Colorado, to one of the fattest states. No, I'm not going to mention which one. But, I was instantly overwhelmed by the massive number of people who were very obese.

So back to the title of this section. Count calories. Calories count. Calories are like money. If you deposit $100 a week into a savings account, and don't withdraw anything, at the end of the year, you will have $5200 in the account. (I'm ignoring interest.) If you put an extra 100 calories a week into your body, at the end of the year, you will about a pound and a quarter heavier, all other things being equal. If you put an extra 100 calories a day into your body – easy to do, a simple slice of cheese is about 90 calories – then at the end of the year you will be about 9 pounds heavier.

Years ago, a presidential candidate ran a successful campaign with the slogan "It's the economy, stupid." It's that simple. It's the calories, chum. You eat and you get them. Exercise and you burn them. It is a lot easier to not eat them than to exercise to burn them. The 350 calorie candy bar that you don't eat saves you three and a half miles of walking. Which is easier? To walk an extra three and a half miles, or to decide to skip the candy bar? Yes, I know, sometimes that candy bar is irresistible. The candy bar people really WANT it to be irresistible. They make money by selling it to you. I'm guessing LOTS of money. Not only that, they go out of their way with subtle advertising. "Snickers satisfies you", and other slogans. Plus, look at the calorie deception in the Nutrition Label. Many times the calories don't sound too bad, until you notice that they count one candy bar as TWO servings. Get real.

Moving the Belt

As you progress, there will be a time (I hope) when your belt gets loose, and you have to buckle it one notch in from where you've been buckling it. HURRAY!!!!!! That is exactly what is supposed to happen. And when it does happen, make up your mind right then and there, that you are NOT going back. Moving the belt is a notable achievement. Make that the new high water mark. And keep working your way down.

Look at this another way. If you have an interest in aviation, or if you have watched a movie or two, you have heard of the term "Point of no Return". But just in case, the "Point of no Return" is that point, in an airplane's travels between its starting point, and its destination, where it no longer has the fuel to make it back to where it took off. It can only continue on towards its destination. This is especially important if flying over an ocean – maybe from Hawaii to San Francisco.

Make that new belt notch, your very own "Point on no Return". Think on it. You can't go back. You can only go forward. Burn that into your consciousness. Not in a terrifying way. But in a celebratory one! You've accomplished something. Keep nudging forward.

Help! I really blew it...

Help. I really blew it...Last night. Yesterday. Last week. Last month. Last **year**. Ok. Let's take a look at this one step at a time.

I really blew it last night.

So, you went on a binge. A really big dinner. A party. A football game. A few too many. Whatever... The good news is that whatever you ate, it's not as bad as it seems. For example, if you ate a whole pound of cheese, it only contains about 1800 calories. This is just a little over a half pound of excess energy (fat). And your digestive system is NOT 100% efficient. If you ate a pound of steak, it is even less of an issue. A 16 oz. steak is about 900 calories. This equates to about a quarter pound of excess energy. Did you over-indulge in alcoholic beverages? Four beers, at about 230 calories each, is only 920 calories, or about a quarter pound. Four glasses of wine, at 140 calories a glass, is only 560 calories, or about one sixth of a pound. And so on. So you see, it is just a blip on the overall downward slope you are travelling. Don't sweat it. Just keep applying the little nudges that are in your arsenal. Don't kick yourself. In fact, just forget it. It's not a big deal.

I really blew it YESTERDAY.

Ok, it happens. Bad day at work. Or at home. Or an old friend is in town and you played all day. Read the paragraph on "I blew it last night.", and apply it to your current situation. You are on a long term, gentle approach. You are headed in the right direction. As they say (whoever "they" are), Rome wasn't built in a day. Neither will it be torn down in a day. Enough said.

I really blew it last week.

So what was the issue? Did you get fired from your job? Did your expected pay raise not come through? Or did your dog die? (or need a $3000 surgery?) Your favorite stock tanked. You got 3 F's on your report card. Ok, I'm out of guesses. But, obviously, something significant happened, and you took refuge in your favorite foods. Or maybe your spouse went out of town on a business trip and you decided to indulge in all the things you couldn't when he/she is with you. Pizza and beer? Steak every night? Chinese take out. Hot dogs and pretzels. WHATEVER. Or, did you go on a business trip with full expenses? Dining out every night with a hefty per diem can certainly pack on the pounds.

So, let's take stock. How much more do you weigh after your week of over-indulgence? A pound? 3 pounds? 5 pounds? I can't imagine it could be any more than that in just one week. In any case, unless you have also invented a time machine in the last week, you are stuck with the fact that you now weigh more than you did last week. What can you do? Simply this: nudge your way down. Would you feel better if you have to say 5 "Our Father"s and 5 "Hail Mary"s? Then do that, too. My point is that you always work from where you are, not from where you wish you were, or where you might have been. The scale doesn't lie. And it doesn't care. And it doesn't hold a grudge. And it doesn't criticize. It just is. Tune in to your goal. Accept the fact that it will take a little longer. Don't get miserable. DON'T panic and start "dieting". And starving. And all that. Just work at the smooth little nudges that will get you to your goal. Maybe it would be good to write some of them on a 3x5 card, or a smaller one that will fit in your billfold. The act of writing things down seems to somehow cement them into your memory. And be glad that you're in the category of the next paragraph. (You aren't are you?)

I really blew it last month.

YOU'VE got to be kidding. A whole month??!! Wow, I am sorry. This signals to me that there has been something major going on in your life. Or you won the lottery and were really celebrating, in which case, how about sending me a million or so? No matter. The idea is the same. Erase from your memory the weight you had a month ago, and put in what you weigh today. There is no magic to this. Perhaps you should re-read the first few chapters so you might remember all the little nudges that you can re-apply. This is not the time to try anything drastic. No starving. Just reorient your thinking back to the strategy of simple little changes that over the long term get you back to an ideal weight.

I really blew it last year.

Well, at least you found the book and are reading it again. I do wonder, just a little, if you really want to bring your weight in line. But, perhaps you had a tour of duty in Belgium. Or, you became the US attaché to Norway and had to entertain dignitaries every weekend for a year. Yes, I'm simply guessing at this point. Thanks for coming back and giving me your vote of confidence. Do read all the other "I really blew it ______________" sections. Now pretend that you are reading the book for the first time, and apply a few nudges this week, a few more next week, and so on. It won't be long until you are in it full swing, without ever DIETING, and on your way to your desired end weight.

The Plateau

Have you ever been hiking? I mean, REAL hiking. In mountains. Ok, if you live in Kansas, or another of the completely flat states, then you might as well skip this chapter. For the rest of you, keep reading...

Hiking up a mountain trail, first of all, is a lot of fun. You are on your way to the top of something. And after an hour or two, and it looks like you are almost there, you reach a flat spot: a plateau. It is lovely. Lots of flowers. Perhaps a small lake. Birds chirping. Deer at the far end. You get the picture. But, you're not at the summit yet. After briefly enjoying the scenery, you move on towards the top. Hold that thought. Because after you have reached the end of the trail, unless it goes in a loop, you come back down the same trail, and hit that plateau again. It is just as lovely in the afternoon light. In some ways, it is even better, because you are on your way down. You've been there before, and you know how far it is to get back to the bottom of the trail. It is relaxing to get there – hiking down a hill is sometimes more strenuous than going uphill. Consequently, you rest a little bit. You look around a bit more than when you were on the way up. You enjoy the sound of the small waterfall at the downward end of the lake/pond. Then, after that breather, you feel refreshed, and head down the path to finish your hike.

Now, let's see how this relates to your downward travels on the weight scale. You are probably going to hit a plateau at some point. You've made it past halfway on your march down to your (ideal) weight goal. It is usually at a weight that is comfortable for you. Maybe a weight that you occupied for a significant time, earlier in life. It might be what you weighed in college. Or just after you married. Or some point in your career. At any rate, it is a place you get sort of stuck. You might hover at one weight for a couple of months. You don't seem to be losing any weight. You've plateaued. (I already said that, didn't I?) WHY? It's really not a mystery. You've relaxed. You know you've made a lot of progress. Your spouse is more interested in you. You feel better about the way you look. Your clothes are looser. You know you can make it the rest of the way. You've proven that. My guess is that you are 30 pounds lighter, with 20 pounds to go. But, the plateau is not the Finish Line.

Getting Unstuck

What to do. Very simply, remind yourself of the things you've been doing to nudge yourself down to where you are. Set a short term goal of perhaps just 5 pounds less than your current weight. In a month. Think about skipping a meal. Look for a few new ways to substitute a lower calorie (but just as tasty) food item for one of your routine snacks/meals. Add an exercise to do daily. Or more likely, restart the things that you have inadvertently dropped. (How many times have you looked at that stack of pennies, but didn't take the time to move them to the other end of the house, one at a time?) Remember, it was about 17 calories a day, over a long period of time, that got you where you were. Nudge down just a bit more each day and you will get unstuck and back on track to the bottom.

Another thing to review is whether all this occurred during the dreaded North American Seasonal Gravity Anomaly. If that is the case, then I urge you to ponder ways to minimize the known effects of that phenomena. After all, it happens every year. Without fail. Have a plan.

Healthful Eating Choices

Yes, this is a chapter you don't want to read. So don't. Skip to the next chapter. I won't be offended.

Still here? Ok, then. Should you be eating more healthfully? OF COURSE! We all should. Are you going to change what you eat, and the way you eat? More than likely, no. You are pretty far into adulthood. You have your likes and dislikes. However, that doesn't mean you can't do a few internet searches, and decide for yourself what food items you might exchange for something just as tasty, but with more health benefits. Am I going to list theme here? NO. There are books, and web sites galore, that can do a much better job than I could ever hope to do. I am a fan of real butter as opposed to margarine. And of real maple syrup vs. that sugary stuff that might have 4% maple syrup in it. Real, whole fruits are clearly better than fruit flavored paste in toaster pop-ups. I'm leery of anything that says "hydrogenated" on the label. Why would I want hydrogen mixed in with my food, anyway? Cereals that have names starting with "Sugar Frosted"? You can't be serious.

Have I made my point? You could go all natural, vegan, raw vegetables, fruits and nuts. You can eat everything out of a can, or eat pre-packaged microwave dinners all the time. Or somewhere in between.

The calorie equation is still the same. If you put more calories into your

body than you burn, you get larger. If you burn more calories than you

consume, you get thinner. You just might live longer on the healthier

foods. And suffer less diseases. (Just my speculation...)

You Are In Control

There was a TV show, back in the '60s that announced at the beginning "There is nothing wrong with your television set. Do not attempt to adjust the picture. We are controlling transmission. If we wish to make it louder, we will bring up the volume. If we wish to make it softer, we will tune it to a whisper. We can reduce the focus to a soft blur, or sharpen it to crystal clarity. We will control the horizontal. We will control the vertical. For the next hour, sit quietly and we will control all that you see and hear. You are about to experience the awe and mystery which reaches from the inner mind to... The Outer Limits."

Well, nothing could be further from the truth, for you. YOU control your own horizontal. YOU control your own vertical. This is YOUR set. Everything is your own decision. Do you want that Super-Jumbe-Extra-Large box of French fries? Then you decide to order it. Do you want the second beer or glass of wine? Then you decide to pour it and drink it. Do you want to lose that next pound, or do you want to gain that next pound? YOU DECIDE. Unless you are in prison and are being force-fed (usually because you are starving yourself in a hunger protest of some sort, so this is sort of nonsensical...), every eating decision, every exercising decision, is yours. Look at that whatever, and overlay it with the number of calories it has, and divide that by 100, which is about 1

mile of walking or running, and decide which way it is going to be. Then

apply all the knowledge and principles you've gain from reading this

book. Nudge. Nudge. Nudge. Compare that to rocket science: $\Delta V = V_e * \ln$

(m_o/m_f) . In my mind, a little nudge is easier to do and understand.

Resisting the Temptation to Shove

Here's the scenario: you are closing in on your target weight. And you've been consistently paring down the pounds. Your goal is only 5, maybe7 pounds away. It is so tempting to go on a 4 day fast, or do one of those "Hollywood" diet drink things, or run 4 miles a day. DON'T!!!!!

Let's go back to the airplane that is descending to a new altitude. Can you imagine what would happen if, when the pilot is 400 feet away from the target altitude, he or she pushes the stick forward suddenly, in order to get there RIGHT NOW?! It would be chaos. Flight attendants would be hurtled into the air. Cups (champagne flutes in First Class, small Styrofoam coffee cups for the rest of us), laptops, small children, and so on, would get scattered all about the cabin. Plus, at the new altitude, the pilot would have to just as quickly pull back on the stick to hold that altitude, pinning everyone into the seat. Obviously, that's not going to happen. The professional pilot gently arrives at the new altitude, and nudges the stick back to level out, and nobody even notices that anything has happened.

It should be the same for you. Simply be patient and persistent. There is no competition. It's not like the 100 meter dash, where the runners lean forward at the last 10th of a second trying to get a nose

ahead of the other runners. You have already won. The fact that you are

closing in on your target weight is testimony to that.

You've Arrived. Welcome to the "New Equilibrium"!

Congratulations! It wasn't that difficult. You are at your "New Equilibrium". You never even went on a diet. You simply applied some common sense to your lifestyle. You can let up on some of the things you have been doing. After all, you don't want to keep losing weight. (Ha Ha!) You don't want to gain it back, either. Just like geo-stationary satellites, you want to stay within your operational box. Probably plus or minus 3 pounds. Keep weighing yourself daily. If you drift up in weight beyond three pounds, gently re-apply the nudges that you know so well. If you drift down beyond three pounds, EAT MORE. The reality is that you can maintain this weight for just about the rest of your life. I'm pretty certain that you have the intelligence to figure out how to stay there quite effortlessly. If not, you at least have all the tools at your disposal from this book. Apply your nudges as necessary, but no more than necessary. You want to simply be at your "New Equilibrium" weight. Whatever you were doing at your old equilibrium weight will probably mostly still work.

Wrapping it up

You've read the book. It wasn't too painful. You have a lot of "nudges" at your fingertips. You know that the easiest thing to do is eat a little less. It is a lot less work than vigorous exercise. And it takes less time. You have a bunch of easy exercises you can do throughout the day. You know that building a little muscle helps nudge up your metabolism, and I think it makes you look better as well.

I'm a fan of making a list. Probably too much of one. My wallet has, at this very moment, about 4 lists in it. There are no doubt some duplicates on those lists. But I don't have to worry about forgetting these things. Make your list of how you are going to do your nudging. Go through the things you eat and pick the things that could work for you. Think about your daily routine and think about where you could add some exercises. (Walking up and down every aisle in the supermarket is so easy!) Then…simply get started. Whether it is a six month effort, a year, two years, or three years, it will be worth it. And (I am mentioning this again…) without dieting. With persistence and patience, you will go from where you are to where you want to be. **NUDGE: The New Equilibrium Diet**